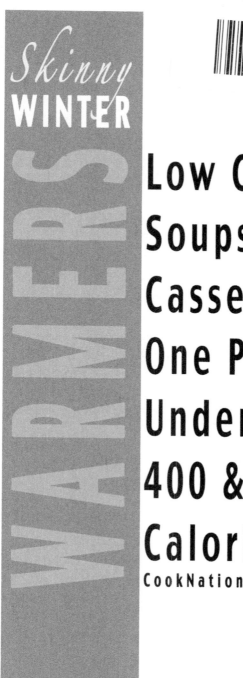

Skinny
WINTER
WARMERS

Low Calorie Soups, Stews, Casseroles & One Pot Meals Under 300, 400 & 500 Calories

CookNation

Skinny Winter Warmers:
Low Calorie Soups, Stews, Casseroles and One Pot
Meals Under 300, 400 & 500 Calories

A Bell & Mackenzie Publication
First published in 2013 by Bell & Mackenzie Publishing
Copyright © Bell & Mackenzie Publishing 2013

ISBN 978-10909855-11-3

A CIP catalogue record of this book is available from the
British Library

Disclaimer
The information and advice in this book is intended as a
guide only. Any individual should independently seek the
advice of a health professional before embarking on a diet.

Some recipes may contain nuts or traces of nuts. Those
suffering from any allergies associated with nuts should
avoid any recipes containing nuts or nut based oils.

Contents

Contents

Contents

Introduction

When the days become shorter, darker and colder and foliage turns to magical autumnal colours, is there anything more comforting than a homemade stew, casserole, one pot or soup to warm the soul?

Traditionally winter warming foods are rich, filling and more often than not, laden with carbs, calories and fats. Many of us become less active in the winter months compared to other parts of the year. We have less daylight hours to stay busy, harsher weather to contend with and a primal instinct to stay inside for longer to keep warm. Combine all these elements and before you know it the winter months can mean you accumulate extra pounds that are difficult to shed.

Hearty winter warming meals needn't be high in calories. With careful preparation and thought you can still enjoy the best in comfort food without worrying about putting on weight. All our Winter Warmer recipes fall below 200, 300, 400 or 500 calories and will help see you through the winter months with your figure intact. Each recipe provides a balanced, nutritious meal serving 4 people so you can feed your family while still keeping check on your own calorie intake.

All the recipes in Skinny Winter Warmers are simple, easy to prepare meals using easily obtainable store cupboard ingredients. Where appropriate we offer alternative ingredients and side serving suggestions to cater to your own tastes.

What This Book Will Do For You

The recipes in this book are all low calorie winter warmer dishes for 4, which make it easier for you to monitor your overall daily calorie intake as well as those you are cooking for. The recommended daily calories are approximately 2000 for women and 2500 for men. Recommended guidelines for children aged 5 to 10 are 1800 calories.

Broadly speaking, by consuming the recommended levels of calories each day you should maintain your current weight. Reducing the number of calories (a calorie deficit) will result in losing weight. This happens because the body begins to use fat stores for energy to make up the reduction in calories, which in turn results in weight loss. We have already counted the calories for each dish making it easy for you to fit this into your daily eating plan whether you want to lose weight, maintain your current figure or are just looking for some great-tasting, comforting, winter warming recipes.

I'm Already On A Diet. Can I Use These Recipes?

Yes of course. All the recipes can be great accompaniments to many of the popular calorie-counting diets. We all know that sometimes dieting can result in hunger pangs, cravings and boredom from eating the same old foods day in and day out. Skinny Winter Warmers provide filling meals which should satisfy you for hours afterwards.

I Am Only Cooking For One. Will This Book Work For Me?

Yes. We would recommend making the family sized meal and storing the rest in single size portions for you to use in the future.

Preparation

All the recipes should take no longer than 10-15 minutes to prepare before you can put in the oven for cooking.
All meat and vegetables should be cut into even

sized pieces. Meat generally cooks faster than vegetables, although root vegetables can take longer, so make sure everything is bite-sized.

All meat should be trimmed of visible fat and the skin removed.

Nutrition
All of the recipes in this collection are balanced low calorie family meals which should keep you feeling full and help you avoid snacking in-between meals.

All Recipes Are A Guide Only
All the recipes in this book are a guide only. You may need to alter quantities and cooking times to suit your own appliances.

We hope you enjoy all the recipes in Skinny Winter Warmers - delicious, hearty, comfort meals... without the calories.

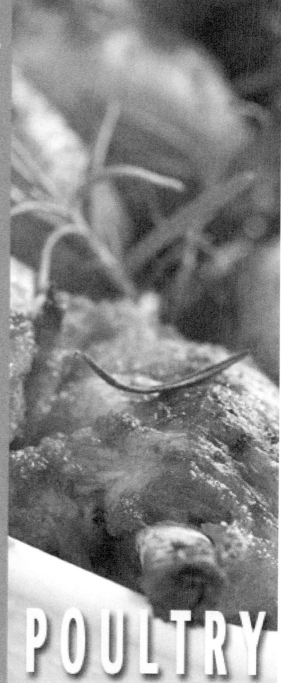

Skinny
WINTER
WARMERS

Soups, Stews
Casseroles &
One Pot Meals
Under 300, 400
& 500 calories

POULTRY

Mild Chicken Coriander Korma

Serves 4

410 CALORIES PER SERVING

Ingredients:

500g/1lb 2oz skinless chicken breast, cubed
380ml/1½ cups tomato passata/sieved tomatoes
1 onion, finely chopped
½ tsp salt
1 tsp brown sugar
1 tbsp mild curry powder
1 tbsp ground almonds
3 tbsp tomato puree/paste
1 tsp each ground garlic, cumin, garam masala, coriander/cilantro & turmeric
60ml/¼ cup coconut milk
200g/7oz basmati rice
2 tbsp freshly chopped coriander/cilantro
Low cal cooking oil spray
Salt & pepper to taste

Method:

• Preheat the oven to 200C/400F/Gas Mark 6.
• Brown the meat for a few minutes in a frying pan with a little low cal spray.
• Add the dried spices, curry powder, onions & tomato puree and gently cook for a minute or two.
• Put in an ovenproof dish and add the tomato passata, sugar, salt and ground almonds.
• Place in the oven and leave to cook for 20-25 minutes or until the chicken is cooked through.
• Meanwhile rinse the rice in a sieve with cold water and cook in a pan of salted boiling water until tender.
• Stir the coconut milk through the curry, serve with the rice and chopped coriander.

You could introduce some sultanas to the recipe during cooking if you want to add some fruity sweetness.

380 CALORIES PER SERVING

Italian Turkey Leek Bake
Serves 4

Method:

• Preheat the oven to 180C/350F/Gas Mark 5.

• First sauté the leeks, garlic and mushrooms in a little low cal spray for a few minutes.

• Add the dried herbs and turkey and cook for a few minutes longer to seal the meat.

• Meanwhile make the creamy sauce by melting the 'butter' in a saucepan, stir in the flour to make a paste and gradually whisk in the milk to make a sauce.

• Continue gently cooking until the sauce thickens a little.

• Stir through the mustard and then combine all the ingredients, except the mashed potato and parsley, in an ovenproof dish.

• Season and top with mashed potato. Cook in the oven for 30-35 minutes or until the turkey is cooked though and piping hot.

• Sprinkle with parsley and serve.

Turkey is a great low-fat versatile meat which works really well in casserole dishes.

Ingredients:

350g/12oz turkey breast, diced
3 leeks, sliced
125g/4oz chestnut mushrooms
2 garlic cloves
2 tsp Italian mixed dried herbs
1 tbsp plain/all purpose flour
1 tbsp low fat 'butter' spread
250ml/1 cup semi skimmed milk
2 tsp dijon mustard
75g/3oz spinach leaves, chopped
2 tbsp freshly chopped flat leaf parsley
150g/5oz tinned cannellini beans, drained
500g/1lb 2oz mashed potato
Low cal cooking oil spray
Salt & pepper to taste

Lahore Chicken Biryani

Serves 4

420 CALORIES PER SERVING

Ingredients:

400g/14oz skinless chicken breast, cubed
370ml/1½ cups tomato passata/sieved tomatoes
1 onion, finely chopped
2 carrots, finely chopped
½ tsp salt
1 tsp brown sugar
3 tbsp tomato puree/paste
75g/3oz frozen peas
1 tsp each ground garlic, cumin, coriander, paprika, garam masala, chilli powder & turmeric
3 tbsp fat free Greek yoghurt
2 tbsp freshly chopped coriander/cilantro
Low cal cooking oil spray
Salt & pepper to taste

Rice Ingredients:

200g/7oz basmati rice
½ onion, finely chopped
¼ tsp ground cinnamon
1 bay leaf
Pinch of saffron threads
1 chicken stock cube
2 tsp sunflower oil

Method:

• Preheat the oven to 200C/400F/Gas Mark 6.
• Brown the meat for a few minutes in a frying pan with a little low cal spray.
• Add the dried spices, onions, carrots & tomato puree and gently cook for a minute or two.
• Put in an ovenproof dish and add the tomato passata, peas, sugar & salt.
• Place in the oven and cook for 20-25 minutes or until the chicken is cooked through.
• Meanwhile rinse the rice in a sieve with cold water. Boil a pan of water and dissolve the cube of chicken stock into it.
• Gently fry the onion and cinnamon for a few minutes in the sunflower oil.
• Add the rice to the onion mix and coat well, transfer contents of frying pan plus the bay leaf and saffron into the boiling stock water and cook until tender. When both the rice and curry are ready, stir the yoghurt through the curry. Combine together and sprinkle with chopped coriander to make a delicious biryani.

Lahore is one of the regions most commonly associated with Biryani, with Chicken being the most popular version.

Turkey Mince Lasagne
Serves 4

Method:

- Preheat the oven to 200C/400F/Gas Mark 6.
- Gently sauté the turkey mince, onion and garlic in a little low cal oil for a few minutes.
- Add the chopped tomatoes, puree, salt & worcestershire sauce and cook for 4-5 minutes.
- Meanwhile mix the ricotta, mozzarella and eggs together. In an ovenproof dish, layer in turn the lasagne sheets, meat and cheese mix, finishing with a layer of meat on top sprinkled with the grated cheddar cheese.
- Cover with foil and cook for 40-50 minutes or until cooked through.
- Remove the foil for the last 10 minutes of cooking to brown the top.
- Sprinkle with chopped parsley & serve.

Ingredients:

500g/1lb 2oz lean minced ground turkey
1 onion, chopped
3 garlic cloves, crushed
400g/14oz tinned chopped tomatoes
2 tbsp tomato puree/paste
2 tsp dried mixed herbs
1 tbsp worcestershire sauce
½ tsp salt
75g/3oz low fat ricotta cheese
75g/3oz low fat mozzarella cheese, grated
75g/3oz low fat cheddar, grated
2 free range eggs, beaten
150g/5oz fresh lasagne sheets
1 tbsp freshly chopped flat leaf parsley
Low cal cooking oil spray
Salt & pepper to taste

Turkey mix is a good lower fat alternative to the traditional beef mince recipe.

15

West Indian Chicken Stew
Serves 4

390 CALORIES PER SERVING

Ingredients:

1 red onion, chopped
500g/1lb 2oz skinless chicken breasts, sliced
300g/11oz plantain, peeled & thinly sliced
3 tsp plain/all-purpose flour
4 garlic cloves, crushed
2 tsp each cayenne pepper, paprika & mustard seeds
4 tsp freshly grated ginger
75h/3oz peas
1 tsp ground cinnamon
250ml/1 cup chicken stock
250ml/1 cup low fat coconut milk
175g/6oz long grain rice
Low cal cooking oil spray
Salt & pepper to taste

Method:

• Preheat the oven to 180C/350F/Gas Mark 5.
• Gently sauté the onion, garlic, dried spices and mustard seeds in a little low cal spray for a few minutes until the onion softens and the mustard seeds begin to pop.
• Stir through the flour and add the hot chicken stock to the pan. Continue stirring for a minute or two.
• Combine all the ingredients, except the coconut milk, in an ovenproof dish.
• Place in the oven and cook for 40-45 minutes or until the chicken is cooked through and the plantain is tender.
• Meanwhile cook the rice in salted boiling water until tender.
• When the chicken is cooked, gently stir through the coconut milk. Season, serve with the boiled rice and pour all the coconut juices over the dish.

Plantain is a starchy banana type vegetable, which must be cooked before eating. You could substitute for sweet potato if you like.

Creamy Chicken & Mini Potato Casserole

Serves 4

Method:

• Preheat the oven to 200C/400F/Gas Mark 6.
• Slice the chicken breasts into strips. Gently sauté the onion and mushrooms in a little low cal oil for a few minutes.
• Add the chicken, stock, paprika and wholegrain mustard to the pan and bring to the boil. Continue stirring for a minute or two while it bubbles away.
• Combine all the ingredients, except the crème fraiche and chopped oregano, in an ovenproof dish.
• Place in the oven and cook for 25-30 minutes or until the chicken is cooked through and the potatoes are tender.
• After cooking, gently stir through the crème fraiche, season and serve with the chopped oregano sprinkled over the top.

Alter the paprika and mustard quantities to suit your own taste.

Ingredients:

500g/1lb 2oz skinless chicken breasts, sliced
2 onions, chopped
1 tbsp wholegrain mustard
1 tsp paprika
250ml/1 cup low fat crème fraiche
200g/7oz small salad potatoes/halved
200g/7oz spinach leaves
2 large portabella mushrooms, sliced
250ml/1 cup chicken stock
1 tbsp freshly chopped oregano
Low cal cooking oil spray
Salt & pepper to taste

Paprika Chicken & Olive Stew
Serves 4

410 CALORIES PER SERVING

Ingredients:

500g/1lb 2oz skinless chicken breasts, sliced
2 onions, chopped
125g/4oz pitted olives, halved
3 tsp smoked paprika
2 tsp dried sage
2 tbsp freshly chopped basil leaves
400g/14oz tinned chopped tomatoes
1 yellow (bell) pepper, sliced
4 garlic cloves, crushed
200g/7oz purple sprouting broccoli, roughly chopped
Low cal cooking oil spray
Salt & pepper to taste

Method:

- Preheat the oven to 200C/400F/Gas Mark 6.
- Gently sauté the onion, sliced pepper, garlic & paprika in a little low cal oil for a few minutes until softened.
- Add the sliced chicken and cook for 3-4 minutes longer.
- Combine all the ingredients, except the chopped basil, in an ovenproof dish.
- Place in the oven and cook for 25-30 minutes or until the chicken is cooked through and the vegetables are tender.
- Season well and serve.

You could also add a handful of chopped capers to this dish if you like.

White Bean Chicken Casserole
Serves 4

Method:

- Preheat the oven to 200C/400F/Gas Mark 6.
- Gently sauté the onion, sliced peppers, garlic & basil in a little low cal oil for a few minutes until softened.
- Add the chopped tomatoes & sliced chicken and cook for 3-4 minutes longer.
- Combine all the ingredients in an ovenproof dish. Place in the oven and cook for 30-40 minutes or until the chicken is cooked through and the vegetables are tender.
- Season well and serve.

Ingredients:

500g/1lb 2oz skinless chicken breasts, sliced
4 shallots, chopped
2 tsp each dried basil
200g/7oz tinned chopped tomatoes
200g/7oz tinned borlotti beans, drained
2 yellow (bell) peppers, sliced
3 garlic cloves, crushed
3 tbsp worcestershire sauce
3 tbsp tomato puree/paste
Low cal cooking oil spray
Salt & pepper to taste

Cannellini beans or butter beans will work well for this dish too.

Chicken & Braised Cabbage
Serves 4

390
CALORIES
PER SERVING

Ingredients:

600g/1lb 5oz skinless chicken breasts, sliced diagonally

200g/7oz French beans

1 red cabbage, shredded

1 red onion, sliced

3 garlic cloves, crushed

250ml/1 cup chicken stock/broth

120ml/½ cup red wine

Low cal cooking oil spray

Salt & pepper to taste

Method:

• Preheat the oven to 180C/350F/Gas Mark 5.
• First braise the cabbage and French beans by adding the chicken stock, shredded cabbage & whole beans to a saucepan and gently cook for 15-20 minutes.
• Meanwhile gently sauté the onions, and garlic in a frying pan with a little low cal spray for a few minutes until soft.
• Add the chicken strips and seal the meat for a few minutes longer.
• Place into an ovenproof dish along with all the other ingredients. Cover and cook in the oven for 20-25 minutes or until the chicken is cooked through and the vegetables are tender.
• Season and serve.

Serve with lots of freshly ground black pepper.

495
CALORIES
PER SERVING

Chicken Stovies
Serves 4

Method:

• Preheat the oven to 200C/400F/Gas Mark 6
• First cook the chicken breasts under a medium grill for 15-25 minutes or until cooked through.
• Shred the meat with two forks and set to one side.
• Meanwhile sauté the pancetta and onions in a frying pan with a little low cal spray for a few minutes.
• Add all the ingredients to an ovenproof dish and combine. Season well, cover and cook in the oven for 40-60 minutes or until the potatoes are tender.
• Ensure the dish doesn't dry up by adding a little more stock during cooking if needed.
• Serve with lots of black pepper.

Ingredients:

500g/1lb 2oz skinless chicken breasts, sliced
450g/1lb desiree potatoes, peeled & cubed
125g/4oz pancetta cubes
2 onions
1 tbsp worcestershire sauce
250ml/1 cup chicken stock
Low cal cooking oil spray
Salt & pepper to taste

Stovies is a classic Scottish dish. This version uses chicken breast, but any leftover roast meat will work.

Italian Chicken & Peppers
Serves 4

360
CALORIES
PER SERVING

Ingredients:

600g/1lb 5oz skinless chicken breasts, sliced diagonally
200g/7oz baby corn, chopped
4 vine ripened tomatoes, chopped
4 red (bell) peppers, sliced
2 red onions, sliced
3 garlic cloves, crushed
1 tsp paprika
1 tsp freshly chopped rosemary
4 tbsp freshly chopped flat leaf parsley
120ml/ ½ cup chicken stock/broth
Low cal cooking oil spray
Salt & pepper to taste

Method:

• Preheat the oven to 180C/350F/Gas Mark 5.
• Gently sauté the onions, peppers and garlic in a frying pan with the paprika and a little low cal spray for a few minutes until soft.
• Add the chicken strips and seal the meat for a few minutes longer.
• Place into an ovenproof dish along with all the other ingredients. Cover and cook in the oven for 30-40 minutes or until the chicken is cooked through and the vegetables are tender.
• Add a little more stock or water during cooking if needed.
• Season and serve.

A mixture of peppers is good in this recipe but avoid the sharp taste of green peppers.

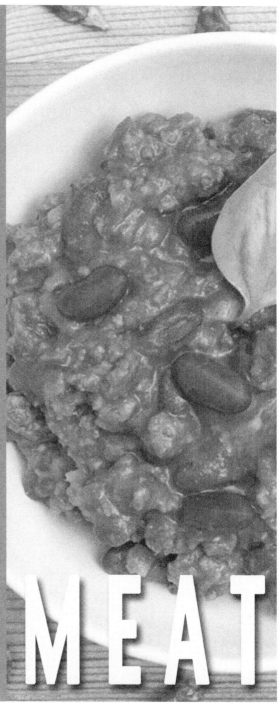

Skinny
WINTER
WARMERS

MEAT

Soups, Stews
Casseroles &
One Pot Meals
Under 300, 400
& 500 calories

Beef & Shallot Casserole
Serves 4-6

350 CALORIES PER SERVING

Ingredients:

1kg/2¼lb beef brisket
450g/1lb shallots, chopped
2 garlic cloves, crushed
1 red onion, chopped
350g/12oz baby carrots, halved lengthways
350g/12oz parsnips, halved lengthways
1 stick celery, chopped
200g/7oz chestnut mushrooms, sliced
250ml/1 cup vegetable stock/broth
1 tbsp each freshly chopped thyme & flat leaf parsley
Low cal cooking oil spray
Salt & pepper to taste

Method:

• Preheat the oven to 140C/275F/Gas Mark 1.
• First trim the beef to get rid of any visible fat then quickly brown the brisket in a frying pan with a little low cal spray, on a high heat for a minute or two.
• Remove from the heat and use the same pan to gently sauté the red onion, garlic, celery, shallots, carrots & parsnips for a few minutes in a little more oil.
• Add all the ingredients, except the chopped parsley, to an ovenproof dish. Cover tightly and leave to cook for 3-3½ hours or until the beef is tender and cooked through.
• At the end of this time remove a small handful of vegetables along with the stock and blend these together in a food processor to make a thick 'gravy'.
• Carve the beef and serve with the cooked vegetables, thick gravy and parsley garnish.

You could alter this recipe to include sweet potatoes and/or chopped tomatoes

Horseradish, Spinach & Beef Steak Casserole

Serves 4

Method:

• Preheat the oven to 140C/275F/Gas Mark 1.
• Quickly brown the steak in a frying pan with a little low cal spray on a high heat for a minute or two.
• Add the onions, carrots & mushrooms and sauté for a few minutes with the beef.
• Stir in the flour and cook for a minute or two longer.
• Stir in the red wine & stock and combine all the ingredients into an ovenproof dish. Season, cover tightly and leave to cook for 2-2½ hours or until the beef is tender and cooked through.

Ingredients:

600g/1lb 5oz lean stewing steak, cubed
2 onions, chopped
2 tbsp plain/all purpose flour
250ml/1 cup beef stock/broth
250ml/1 cup red wine
125g/4oz carrots, chopped
125g/4oz spinach leaves
2 tbsp horseradish sauce
200g/7oz chestnut mushrooms
1 tbsp freshly chopped oregano
Low cal cooking oil spray
Salt & pepper to taste

Shop-bought horseradish sauce is the perfect 'cheat' ingredient for this dish and adds a little 'kick' to the meal.

Beef, Tomato & Red Onion Stew
Serves 4

370
CALORIES
PER SERVING

Ingredients:

600g/1lb 5oz lean stewing steak, cubed
2 red onions, cut into wedges
2 tbsp tomato puree/paste
400g/14oz tinned chopped tomatoes
400g/14oz carrots, chopped
2 garlic cloves, crushed
2 tsp dried rosemary
4 large portabella mushrooms, sliced
Low cal cooking oil spray
Salt & pepper to taste

Method:

• Preheat the oven to 150C/300F/Gas Mark 2.
• Quickly brown the steak in a frying pan with a little low cal spray on a high heat for a minute or two.
• Add the red onions, carrots, mushrooms, garlic & rosemary and sauté for a few minutes along with the beef.
• Stir in the chopped tomatoes bring to the boil and combine all the ingredients into an ovenproof dish. Season, cover tightly and leave to cook for 1½-2 hours or until the beef is tender and cooked through.

Leave to cook uncovered for a little longer if you want to reduce the dish and create a thicker sauce.

420 CALORIES PER SERVING

Sundried Tomato Cottage Pie
Serves 4

Method:

• Preheat the oven to 200C/400F/Gas Mark 6
• Quickly brown the mince in a frying pan with a little low cal spray on a high heat for a minute or two.
• Add the onions, carrots, mushrooms, celery & garlic and gently sauté for a few minutes along with the mince.
• Stir in the sundried tomato paste chopped tomatoes, stock and mixed herbs.
• Season, simmer for 10 minutes and then combine all the ingredients, except the potatoes & milk, into an ovenproof dish.
• Meanwhile make the mash by cooking the potatoes in salted boiling water until tender.
• Mash well and add a splash of milk until smooth. Use the mash to cover the cooked mince in the ovenproof dish. Place in the oven and leave to cook for 30-40 minutes, or until the beef is tender and cooked through.

Ingredients:

450g/1lb lean, ground/minced beef
1 onion, chopped
200g/7oz carrots, chopped
125g/4oz mushrooms, sliced
2 sticks celery, chopped
2 tbsp sundried tomato puree/paste
200g/7oz tinned chopped tomatoes
1 garlic clove, crushed
2 tsp dried mixed herbs
60ml/¼ cup beef stock/broth
900g/2lb desiree potatoes, peeled & cubed
Splash of milk
Low cal cooking oil spray
Salt & pepper to taste

You could add some pre-soaked red lentils to this dish if you wanted to make it even heartier.

Mexican Beef & Bean Chilli

Serves 4

420 CALORIES PER SERVING

Ingredients:

300g/11oz lean, ground/ minced beef
1 onion, chopped
200g/7oz carrots, finely chopped
2 sticks celery, chopped
2 tbsp tomato puree/paste
2 red chillies, deseeded and finely chopped
1 tsp each ground cumin, paprika and coriander/ cilantro
1 tsp brown sugar
200g/7oz tinned chopped tomatoes
400g/14oz tinned mixed beans, drained
2 garlic cloves, crushed
60ml/¼ cup beef stock/ broth
2 tbsp freshly chopped coriander/cilantro
Low cal cooking oil spray
Salt & pepper to taste

Method:

• Preheat the oven to 200C/400F/Gas Mark 6
• Quickly brown the mince in a frying pan with a little low cal spray on a high heat for a minute or two.
• Add the onions, carrots, celery, ground spices & garlic and gently sauté for a few minutes along with the mince.
• Stir in the tomato paste, chopped tomatoes, stock, beans and sugar.
• Season, simmer for 10 minutes and then combine all the ingredients, except the chopped coriander/cilantro, into an ovenproof dish.
• Place in the oven, cover and leave to cook for 20 minutes, or until the beef is tender and cooked through.

Leave to cook uncovered for a little longer if you want to reduce further and create a thicker sauce.

Traditional Beef Stew
Serves 4

Method:

- Preheat the oven to 180C/350F/Gas Mark 5
- Place the beef in a plastic bag with the flour and shake well to cover the meat, then quickly brown the beef in a frying pan with a little low cal spray.
- Remove the beef and gently sauté the bacon, onions, parsnips, garlic, carrots and mushrooms in a little low cal spray for a few minutes.
- Season and add all the other ingredients, except the fresh basil, to the pan. Stir well, bring to the boil and place in an ovenproof dish. Cover tightly and leave to cook in the oven for 40-60 minutes or until the beef is tender & cooked through.
- Remove the lid for the last 10 minutes of cooking to reduce the liquid if needed.
- Serve with the basil sprinkled on top.

Use the best quality stewing steak you can get and feel free to substitute stock instead of red wine.

Ingredients:

**600g/1lb 5oz lean stewing steak, trimmed and cubed
1 tbsp plain/all-purpose flour
125g/4oz lean, back bacon
1 tbsp worcestershire sauce
1 onion, chopped
2 carrots, chopped
2 parsnips, chopped
4 cloves garlic, crushed
125g/4oz mushrooms, sliced
1 tsp each freshly chopped thyme & oregano
120ml/½ cup red wine
500ml/2 cups beef stock/ broth
2 tbsp freshly chopped basil
Low cal cooking oil spray
Salt & pepper to taste**

Cabbage & Corned Beef Hash Bake

Serves 4

493 CALORIES PER SERVING

Ingredients:

400g/14oz lean corned beef, cubed
450g/1lb potatoes, peeled and cut into small cubes
200g/7oz chopped white cabbage
75g/3oz peas
1 carrot, finely chopped
1 onion, sliced
1 tbsp worcestershire sauce
Pinch crushed chilli flakes
120ml/½ cup beef stock/broth
Low cal cooking oil spray
Salt & pepper to taste

Method:

• Preheat the oven to 200C/400F/Gas Mark 6
• Gently sauté the onions, cabbage, carrots and potatoes in a little low-cal spray for 8-10 minutes.
• Season well and combine all the ingredients in an ovenproof dish. Place in the oven and cook for 40-50 minutes or until the vegetables are tender and the stock is absorbed.

Alter the chilli flake and worcestershire sauce quantities to suit your own taste.

430 CALORIES PER SERVING

Baked Bean & Sausage Bake
Serves 4

Method:

• Preheat the oven to 200C/400F/Gas Mark 6

• Brown the sausage in a frying pan with the onions and a little low cal cooking oil for a few minutes and then slice the sausages into 1cm/½ inch slices.

• Combine all the other ingredients in an ovenproof dish and season. Place in the oven and cook for 30-40 minutes or until the sausages are cooked through, the vegetables are tender and the stock is absorbed.

Ingredients:

8 lean pork sausages
600g/1lb 5oz tinned baked beans
400g/14oz tinned chopped tomatoes
1 onion, chopped
2 carrots, finely chopped
1 tbsp tomato puree/paste
1 tsp brown sugar
1 tsp dijon mustard
60ml/¼ cup vegetable stock
Low cal cooking oil spray
Salt & pepper to taste

This is a super-simple suppertime meal which is always really popular with children.

31

Northern Soul Hotpot

Serves 4

470 CALORIES PER SERVING

Ingredients:

500g/1lb 2oz lean lamb
fillet, cubed
2 onions, chopped
4 carrots, chopped
1 tbsp plain/all-purpose
flour
1 tbsp worcestershire
sauce
500ml/2 cups lamb stock/
broth
1 tbsp sundried tomato
puree/paste
2 garlic cloves, crushed
1 bay leaf
1 tsp dried rosemary
2 tbsp freshly chopped
thyme
400g/14oz potatoes,
peeled & thinly sliced
Low cal cooking oil spray
Salt & pepper to taste

*The sundried tomato
paste in this dish
adds a different taste
dimension. Feel free to
substitute with regular
tomato puree if you
prefer.*

Method:

• Preheat the oven to 180C/350F/Gas
Mark 5.
• Brown the lamb in a frying pan
with a little low cal cooking spray for
a few minutes and then place in an
ovenproof dish.
• Put to one side and gently sauté the
carrots and onion in the same pan for
a few minutes using a little more oil if
needed.
• Add the flour and stir well, pour
in the stock, thyme, rosemary,
sundried tomato puree, bay leaf &
worcestershire sauce and bring to the
boil.
• Add the contents of the pan to the
ovenproof dish and stir. Arrange the
potato slices over the top.
• Season well, spray with cooking oil
and cover with foil. Place in the oven
and cook for 40-60 minutes or until the
lamb is cooked through and the potato
slices are tender.
• Remove the foil cover for the last
10 minutes of cooking to brown the
potatoes.

390 CALORIES PER SERVING

BBQ Sauce Pain à la Viande
Serves 4

Method:

• Preheat the oven to 180C/350F/Gas Mark 5.

• Gently brown the beef in a frying pan with a little low cal cooking spray and set to one side.

• In the same pan sauté the onions and sliced peppers for a few minutes.

• Combine all the ingredients, except the BBQ sauce, in an ovenproof dish.

• Season and cook in the oven for 30-40 minutes or until the beef is cooked through and the liquid has reduced down to thick sauce.

• Load the mince into the hot-dog rolls, add the BBQ sauce and serve.

Ingredients:

450g/1lb lean, ground/ minced minced beef
300g/11oz tinned chopped tomatoes
1 onion, chopped
1 red (bell) pepper, chopped
1 tsp mild powder
½ tsp each garlic powder, mustard powder & paprika
1 tsp soy sauce
1 tsp worcestershire sauce
2 tbsp BBQ sauce
4 wholemeal, soft, hot-dog rolls
Salt & pepper to taste
Low cal cooking oil spray

This is a Canadian version of the classic American dish 'Sloppy Joe'. Don't worry about getting messy – remember the joy is in the eating not the cleaning up!

Red Onion Toad In The Hole
Serves 4

350 CALORIES PER SERVING

Ingredients:

8 thick, low-fat pork sausages
125g/4oz plain/all-purpose flour
2 free range eggs
250ml/1 cup semi skimmed milk
2 tsp dijon mustard
½ tsp each of dried thyme and rosemary
1 red onion, thinly sliced into half moons
400g/14oz tinned baked beans
Low cal cooking oil spray
Salt & pepper to taste

Method:

• Preheat the oven to 180C/350F/Gas Mark 5.
• Pierce the sausages and put in an ovenproof dish with a little low cal spray. Cook for 8-12 minutes or until the sausages are browned.
• Add the onions for the last 6 minutes of cooking so that they begin to tenderize.
• Meanwhile make up the batter by sifting the flour into a bowl. Beat the eggs into the flour and gradually add the milk, beating all the time to create a smooth batter. Add the dried herbs, mustard and seasoning.
• Split the cooked sausages lengthways and arrange, along with onions, in the ovenproof dish.
• Pour the batter over the top and cook for a further 25-35 minutes or until the batter is golden brown and puffed up.
• Heat the baked beans in a saucepan and serve with the toad in the hole.

Toad In The Hole is a traditional, fun, family favourite. You can always replace the red onion with regular onion if you prefer.

Aromatic Moroccan Lamb & Peach One Pot

Serves 4

Method:

- Preheat the oven to 180C/350F/Gas Mark 5
- Gently sauté the onion, garlic & spices in a little low cal spray for a few minutes until softened.
- Add the chopped tomatoes & cubed lamb and cook for 3-4 minutes longer.
- Combine all the ingredients, except the chopped parsley, in an ovenproof dish. Place in the oven, cover and leave to cook for 40-50 minutes or until the lamb is tender and cooked through.
- Season well and serve with the chopped parsley sprinkled over the top.

Ingredients:

400g/14oz lean lamb fillet, cubed
2 onions, chopped
2 tsp each ground cumin & coriander/cilantro
1 tsp each ground cinnamon & chilli powder
½ tsp ground nutmeg
4 ripe peaches, stoned and cut into wedges
400g/14oz tinned chopped tomatoes
400g/14oz tinned chickpeas, drained
4 garlic cloves, crushed
3 tbsp worcestershire sauce
3 tbsp tomato puree/paste
2 tbsp freshly chopped flat leaf parsley
Low cal cooking oil spray
Salt & pepper to taste

You can also use tinned peaches in this recipe if you like.

Aubergine Topped Lamb Moussaka
Serves 4

Ingredients:

400g/14oz lean ground
lamb mince
4 small aubergines/
eggplants, halved and
thinly sliced
2 onions, chopped
1 tsp each ground
cinnamon & all spice
2 tsp each oregano &
thyme
2 x 400g/14oz tins
chopped tomatoes
3 garlic cloves, crushed
500ml/2 cups fat free
Greek yoghurt
200g/7oz low fat grated
cheddar cheese
3 tbsp tomato puree/paste
2 tbsp freshly chopped
basil
Low cal cooking oil spray
Salt & pepper to taste

Method:

• Preheat the oven to 180C/350F/Gas
Mark 5.
• Gently sauté the onion, garlic,
aubergines & spices in a little low cal oil
for a few minutes until softened.
• Add the chopped tomatoes, puree &
lamb mince and cook for 3-4 minutes
longer. (you might find it helpful to
sauté the aubergine slices in a separate
pan but you don't have to).
• Place all the ingredients, except the
chopped basil, yoghurt & cheese, in an
ovenproof dish layering the aubergine
slices on top.
• Meanwhile very gently heat the
yoghurt and cheese together in a
saucepan and, when combined,
carefully pour into the ovenproof dish.
• Place in the oven and leave to cook
for 35-40 minutes or until the lamb is
tender and cooked through.
• Season well and serve with the
chopped basil sprinkled over the top.

*This recipe uses aubergine
slices rather than potato slices
for the moussaka topping.*

Ham, Leek & Cheddar Cheese Bake
Serves 4

Method:

- Preheat the oven to 200C/400F/Gas Mark 6.
- Gently sauté the garlic, potatoes & leek in a little low cal spray for a few minutes until softened.
- Gently heat the 'butter' in a saucepan and add the flour, stirring continuously to create a roux.
- Slowly add the milk and carry on stirring to prevent lumps. Warm through until the sauce thickens a little.
- Combine all the ingredients in an ovenproof dish and sprinkle the breadcrumbs on top. Place in the oven and cook for 15-20 minutes or until the vegetables are tender.
- Season well and serve.

Ingredients:

4 tsp low-cal 'butter' spread
4 tsp plain/all-purpose flour
500ml/2 cups semi skimmed milk
400g/14oz desiree potatoes, peeled & cubed
125g/4oz grated low fat mature cheddar cheese
1 tbsp dijon mustard
4 leeks, sliced
400g/14oz lean cooked ham, chopped
125g/4oz fresh breadcrumbs
4 garlic cloves, crushed
4 tbsp freshly chopped parsley
300g/11oz tenderstem broccoli, roughly chopped
Low cal cooking oil spray
Salt & pepper to taste

Make fresh breadcrumbs by placing a slice or two of brown bread in a food processor and pulsing for a few seconds.

Sirloin Stroganoff & Rice
Serves 4

380 CALORIES PER SERVING

Ingredients:

450g/1lb lean sirloin steak, cut into fine strips
2 tsp lemon juice
4 shallots, chopped
1 tsp each dried rosemary & paprika
3 large portabella mushrooms, sliced
2 garlic cloves, crushed
1 tsp dijon mustard
120ml/½ cup beef stock
250ml/1 cup low fat crème fraiche
300g/11oz long grain rice
2 tbsp freshly chopped flat leaf parsley
Low cal cooking oil spray
Salt & pepper to taste

Method:

- Preheat the oven to 200C/400F/Gas Mark 6.
- Gently sauté the shallots, garlic & mushrooms in a little low cal oil for a few minutes.
- Add the steak and cook for 3-4 minutes longer. Place all the ingredients, except the rice, lemon juice and parsley, in an ovenproof dish and combine well. Cook in the oven for 15-20 minutes or until the sauce is creamy & the steak is tender and cooked through (add a little more crème fraiche or stock if needed).
- Meanwhile cook the rice in salted boiling water until tender.
- Season the steak well and stir in the lemon juice.
- Serve with the stroganoff piled on top of a bed of rice and the parsley sprinkled on top.

Cut the steak as thinly as possible. Try putting it in the freezer for half an hour before slicing and you'll find it easier to cut finely.

Chorizo & Pepper Stew
Serves 4

Method:

• Preheat the oven to 200C/400F/Gas Mark 6.
• Gently sauté the onion, sliced peppers, garlic & herbs in a little low cal oil for a few minutes until softened.
• Add the sausages and chorizo and cook for 3-4 minutes longer. Slice the chorizo & sausages into thick rounds.
• Combine all the ingredients in an ovenproof dish and cook for 25-30 minutes or until the sausages are cooked through and the kidney beans are tender.
• Season well and serve.

Ingredients:

200g/7oz lean pork sausages
200g/7oz uncooked chorizo sausages
2 red onions, chopped
4 red (bell) peppers, sliced
3 tsp each mixed dried herbs & smoked paprika
400g/14oz tinned chopped tomatoes
400g/14oz tin red kidney beans, drained
4 garlic cloves, crushed
2 tbsp worcestershire sauce
3 tbsp tomato puree/paste
Low cal cooking oil spray
Salt & pepper to taste

Use uncooked chorizo sausage for this dish rather than the salami-style cured chorizo.

Sweet Potato Pork & Apple Casserole
Serves 4

320
CALORIES
PER SERVING

Ingredients:

500g/1lb 2oz pork loin
steaks, thinly sliced
250ml/1 cup pure apple
juice
4 golden delicious apples
(or similar), peeled &
chopped
8 garlic cloves, crushed
3 large portabella
mushrooms, sliced
120ml/½ cup soured
cream
300g/11oz sweet potatoes,
peeled and cut into
matchsticks
Low cal cooking oil spray
Salt & pepper to taste

Method:

• Preheat the oven to 200C/400F/Gas
Mark 6.
• Gently sauté the sliced pork, chopped
apples, sweet potatoes, garlic and
mushrooms in a little low cal oil for a
few minutes until softened.
• Stir through the apple juice & crème
fraiche and combine everything in an
ovenproof dish.
• Place in the oven and cook for 20-25
minutes or until the pork is cooked
through and the sweet potatoes are
tender.

*You could use butternut squash
instead of sweet potatoes if you
prefer.*

Pork, Broccoli & Butternut Squash Stew
Serves 4

Method:

• Preheat the oven to 180C/350F/Gas Mark 5.
• Season the pork tenderloin. Spray with a little low cal cooking oil and quickly brown in a frying pan for a few minutes.
• Place in an ovenproof dish with all the other ingredients and cover tightly. Cook for 45-50 minutes or until the pork is cooked through and the squash is tender.
• Remove the pork and cut into thick slices. Arrange on the plate with the broccoli and squash to the side.
• Pour the juices over the top of the pork and serve.

Ingredients:

500g/1lb 2oz piece of pork tenderloin
180ml/¾ cup chicken stock
60ml/¼ cup fresh orange juice
4 garlic cloves, crushed
4 tbsp freshly chopped sage
300g/11oz butternut squash, peeled & cut into small cubes
200g/7oz tenderstem broccoli, chopped
Low cal cooking oil spray
Salt & pepper to taste

Dried sage will do fine if you don't have any fresh sage to hand.

Chocolate & Cinnamon Chilli
Serves 4

Ingredients:

Low cal cooking oil spray
500g/1lb 2oz lean,
minced/ground beef
1 cinnamon stick
1 tsp each ground cumin &
chilli powder
1 ½ tbsp cocoa powder
4 carrots, cut into batons
2 onions, chopped
200g/7oz ripe tomatoes,
chopped
4 garlic cloves, crushed
1 tbsp dried basil
2 tbsp tomato puree/paste
250ml/1 cup beef stock
300g/11oz long grain rice
Salt & pepper to taste

Method:

• Preheat the oven to 200C/400F/Gas Mark 6.
• Gently sauté the onion, garlic, spices & herbs in a little low cal spray for a few minutes until softened.
• Add all the other ingredients, except the cinnamon stick, and cook for 4-5 minutes longer.
• Combine well in an ovenproof dish, add the cinnamon stick and cook in the oven for 30-40 minutes or until the mince is cooked through and the stock is absorbed.
• Meanwhile cook the rice in salted boiling water until tender.
• Remove the cinnamon stick and serve the chilli piled on top of the rice.

Use less chilli powder if you don't want the dish to have a 'kick'.

386 CALORIES PER SERVING

Sausage & Lentil Stew

Serves 4

Method:

• Preheat the oven to 180C/350F/Gas Mark 5

• Gently sauté the sausages, onion, peppers, garlic & tomatoes in a little low cal oil for a few minutes.

• When the sausages are sealed, slice into 1cm/½ inch thick rounds. Add all the ingredients to an ovenproof dish and season well.

• Cover with foil, place in the oven and leave to cook for 30-35 minutes or until the sausages are cooked and the lentils are tender.

• Add a little water during cooking if you find the lentils are drying up the dish.

It is especially good to use a really meaty farmhouse-type sausage for this dish.

Ingredients:

8 low fat pork sausages
300g/7oz boneless, skinless cod fillets, cut into chunks
1 onion, chopped
1 red (bell) pepper, sliced
3 garlic cloves, crushed
400g/14oz tinned red kidney beans, drained
200g/7oz vine ripened tomatoes, chopped
250ml/1 cup tomato passatta/sieved tomatoes
125g/4oz red lentils
3 carrots, sliced
2 tsp dried mixed herbs
1 tsp paprika
1 tbsp freshly chopped flat leaf parsley
Low cal cooking oil spray
Salt & pepper to taste

Beef Tagine
Serves 4

465 CALORIES PER SERVING

Ingredients:

600g/1lb 5oz lean stewing steak
1 tsp each ground turmeric, cumin, coriander/cilantro & paprika
2 onions, chopped
1 tbsp plain/all purpose flour
1 red chilli, deseeded and finely chopped
450g/1lb sweet potatoes, peeled & thinly sliced
500ml/2 cups beef stock/broth
3 carrots, chopped
3 tbsp freshly chopped flat leaf parsley
Low cal cooking oil spray
Salt & pepper to taste

Method:

• Preheat the oven to 180C/350F/Gas Mark 5
• Place the beef in a plastic bag with the flour and shake well to cover the meat.
• Quickly brown the beef in a frying pan in a little low cal spray for a few minutes.
• Add all the ingredients, except the parsley, to an ovenproof dish and layer the sweet potato slices on top to cover.
• Season well, place in the oven and cook for 1–1½ hours or until the meat & vegetables are tender. Add a little more stock during cooking if needed.
• Take the foil off and increase the heat for the last 10 minutes to brown the potatoes.
• Sprinkle with parsley and serve

A little lemon zest sprinkled over the top during serving gives the dish a fresh 'lift.'

465 CALORIES PER SERVING

Lamb Fillet & Broad Bean Stew
Serves 4

Method:

• Preheat the oven to 180C/350F/Gas Mark 5
• Quickly brown the lamb in a little low cal spray.
• Add all the ingredients, except the chopped coriander, broad beans and spinach, to an ovenproof dish.
• Season well, place in the oven and cook for 1–1½ hours or until the meat & vegetables are tender.
• Add the broad beans and spinach for the last 30 minutes of cooking and ensure the dish doesn't dry up by adding a little more stock during cooking if needed.
• Remove the bay leaf, sprinkle with chopped coriander and serve.

Ingredients:

500g/1lb 2oz lean lamb fillet, cubed
4 garlic cloves, crushed
1 tsp each coriander/ cilantro & paprika
2 onions, chopped
1 tbsp plain/all purpose flour
200g/7oz fresh shelled broad beans
200g/7oz spinach leaves
1 tbsp freshly chopped coriander/cilantro
120ml/½ cup lamb stock
1 bay leaf
Low cal cooking oil spray
Salt & pepper to taste

Adding the spinach and broad beans towards the end of the cooking time means these vegetables retain their form.

Pork & Cider Casserole
Serves 4

Ingredients:

500g/1lb 2oz pork
tenderloin, cubed
4 garlic cloves, crushed
125g/4oz dried apricots,
chopped
250ml/1 cup dry cider
250ml/1 cup chicken stock
2 tbsp plain/all purpose
flour
2 onions, chopped
2 parsnips, very finely
chopped
2 celery stalks, chopped
400g/14oz tinned flageolet
beans, drained
1 tbsp freshly chopped
parsley
Low cal cooking oil spray
Salt & pepper to taste

Method:

• Preheat the oven to 180C/350F/Gas
Mark 5
• Place the cubed pork in a plastic bag
with the flour and shake well to cover
the meat.
• Quickly brown the pork in a frying
pan in a little low cal spray for a few
minutes.
• Add all the ingredients, except the
chopped parsley, to an ovenproof dish.
• Season well, place in the oven and
cook for 1-1½ hours or until the meat &
vegetables are tender.
• Ensure the dish doesn't dry up
by adding a little more stock during
cooking if needed.
• Sprinkle with chopped parsley and
serve

*Apple juice rather than cider
will work well in this recipe too.*

415 CALORIES PER SERVING

Smokey Bacon Bean Stew
Serves 4

Method:

• Preheat the oven to 140C/275F/Gas Mark 1.
• Cook the bacon and brown the sausages in a frying pan with a little low cal spray for a few minutes along with the carrots and onions.
• Add all the ingredients to an ovenproof dish. Season well, place in the oven and cook for 3-4 hours or until the meat, beans & vegetables are tender.
• Ensure the dish doesn't dry up by adding a little more stock during cooking if needed.

Ingredients:

200g/7oz dried cannellini beans
150g/5oz smoked back bacon
200g/7oz lean sausages
6 garlic cloves, peeled
250ml/1 cup red wine
250ml/1 cup chicken stock/broth
2 tbsp freshly chopped thyme
1 onion, chopped
2 carrots, finely chopped
Low cal cooking oil spray
Salt & pepper to taste

Slow cooking this dish really blends the flavours together in this lovely thick stew.

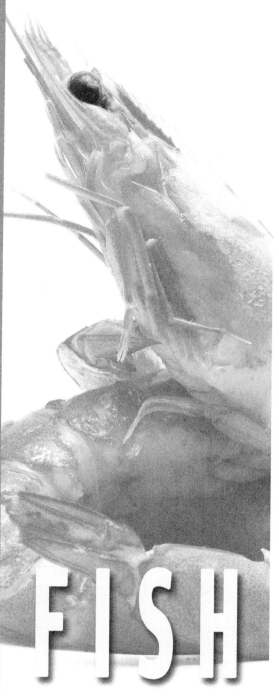

Skinny
WINTER
WARMERS

Soups, Stews
Casseroles &
One Pot Meals
Under 300, 400
& 500 calories

FISH

Hearty Fish Pie
Serves 4

470 CALORIES PER SERVING

Ingredients:

225g/8oz boneless, skinless salmon fillets
225g/8oz boneless, skinless haddock fillets
800g/1lb 11oz desiree potatoes, peeled and cubed
75g/3oz peas
75g/3oz sweetcorn
125g/4oz low fat mature cheddar cheese, grated
2 carrots, finely chopped
25g/1oz low fat 'butter' spread
1 tbsp plain/all-purpose flour
500ml/2 cups skimmed milk
1 tsp wholegrain mustard
2 tbsp freshly chopped flat leaf parsley
Salt & pepper to taste

Feel free to use alternative fish in this recipe. Any meaty white fish is good with the salmon.

Method:

• Preheat the oven to 200C/400F/Gas Mark 6.
• Place the fish in a pan and cover with milk. Gently poach for 8-10 minutes until the fish is cooked and flakes easily with a fork.
• Remove the fish from the pan and reserve the milk. Place the cooked fish, sweetcorn, carrots & peas in an ovenproof dish.
• Meanwhile, cook the potatoes in salted boiling water until tender. When they are ready, drain and mash using a splash of the fishy milk.
• Gently melt the low fat spread in a pan and stir through the flour. When you have made a roux (paste) begin adding the reserved fishy milk and continue stirring.
• The sauce will thicken after a minute or two then add the mustard and cheese.
• Remove from the heat and pour onto the fish and vegetables in the ovenproof dish. Cover with the smooth mash, place in the oven and cook for 30-40 minutes or until the vegetables are tender and the fish is piping hot.
• Serve with the chopped parsley sprinkled over the top.

Pollack Gratin
Serves 4

Method:

• Preheat the oven to 200C/400F/Gas Mark 6.
• Gently sauté the mushrooms, garlic, onions & anchovy paste together in a little low cal spray for a few minutes.
• Add the chopped tomatoes and sliced fish fillets and gently warm through.
• Place in an ovenproof dish and sprinkle with the breadcrumbs & parmesan. Cook for 25-30 minutes or until the fish is properly cooked through.
• Serve with the rocket salad and lemon wedges.

Ingredients:

500g/1lb 2oz boneless, skinless pollack fillets, sliced
4 garlic cloves, crushed
2 onions, chopped
150g/5oz fresh breadcrumbs
1 tbsp grated parmesan cheese
4 tbsp freshly chopped flat leaf parsley
4 large portabella mushrooms, sliced
400g/7oz tinned chopped tomatoes
1 tbsp anchovy paste
200g/7oz rocket leaves
2 lemons, cut into wedges
Low cal cooking oil spray
Salt & pepper to taste

Make fresh breadcrumbs by placing a slice or two of brown bread in a food processor and pulsing for a few seconds.

Salmon & Asparagus Bake
Serves 4

260 CALORIES PER SERVING

Ingredients:

4 thick skinless, boneless salmon fillets - each weighing 125g/4oz
4 tsp runny honey
2 tbsp soy sauce
5 tbsp water
2 tsp sesame oil
2 lemons, cut into wedges
300g/11oz asparagus spears
125g/4oz mangetout
75g/3oz mature cheddar cheese, grated
Salt & pepper to taste

Method:

• Preheat the oven to 200C/400F/Gas Mark 6.
• Mix together the honey, soy sauce, water and sesame oil.
• Place the salmon fillets, asparagus and mangetout in an ovenproof dish and gently combine well with the oil & honey mix.
• Cook for 20-25 minutes or until the salmon fillets are properly cooked through and the vegetables are tender.
• Sprinkle the cheese over the asparagus to melt 2-3 mins before the end of cooking.
• Serve with lemon wedges on the side.

Feel free to experiment with seasonal veg such as kale or pak choi.

Tuna & Egg Noodle Casserole
Serves 4

Method:

- Preheat the oven to 200C/400F/Gas Mark 6.
- Gently sauté the onion in a little low cal spray for a few minutes until soft.
- Meanwhile cook the egg noodles in salted boiling water until tender.
- Combine all the ingredients really well in an ovenproof dish.
- Season, place in the oven and cook for 20-25 minutes or until piping hot.

Ingredients:

3 onions, chopped
500g/1lb 2oz tinned tuna, drained
200g/7oz peas
350g/12oz fine egg noodles
400g/14oz tinned chopped tomatoes
1 tsp crushed chilli flakes
3 tbsp sundried tomato puree/paste
Low cal cooking oil spray
Salt & pepper to taste

Tuna and noodle casserole is a classic one-pot meal in the US. This version uses a tomato base but you could use a creamy base by substituting with condensed mushroom soup.

Philadelphia Seafood Bake
Serves 4

430 CALORIES PER SERVING

Ingredients:

150g/5oz fresh
breadcrumbs
200g/7oz small peeled
prawns
200g/7oz boneless cod fish
fillets, cut into chunks
200g/7oz boneless smoked
haddock fillets, cut into
chunks
200g/7oz spinach,
chopped
200g/7oz tender kale,
roughly chopped
200g/7oz sweetcorn
250ml/1 cup milk
4 tbsp low fat Philadelphia
cream cheese
2 lemons, cut into wedges
Salt & pepper to taste

Method:

• Preheat the oven to 200C/400F/Gas
Mark 6.
• Gently heat the milk and cream
cheese in a saucepan to make a creamy
sauce.
• Carefully combine all the ingredients
in an ovenproof dish, season and
sprinkle the breadcrumbs on top.
• Place in the oven and cook for 35-40
minutes or until the seafood is properly
cooked through and the vegetables are
tender.
• Serve with lemon wedges on the
side.

*Make fresh breadcrumbs by
placing a slice or two of brown
bread in a food processor and
pulsing for a few seconds.*

Anchovy, Cod & Tomato Stew
Serves 4

Method:

• Preheat the oven to 200C/400F/Gas Mark 6
• Gently sauté the onion, anchovy fillets & garlic in a little low cal oil for a few minutes until the anchovy fillets begin to break up.
• Add all the ingredients to an ovenproof dish and season well. Cover with foil and leave to cook for 30-35 minutes or until the seafood is properly cooked through.

Ingredients:

300g/7oz small peeled prawns
300g/7oz boneless, skinless cod fillets, cut into chunks
3 onions, chopped
3 garlic cloves, crushed
400g/14oz tinned chopped tomatoes
6 small anchovy fillets in oil, drained
1 tbsp tomato puree/paste
3 tbsp freshly chopped basil
½ tsp crushed chilli flakes
2 bay leaves
Salt & pepper to taste

It's fine to use any combination of seafood you prefer in this dish, alter the amount of chilli flakes to suit your own taste.

Monkfish Creole & Noodle Stew

Serves 4

330 CALORIES PER SERVING

Ingredients:

500g/1lb 2oz skinless, boneless monkfish fillets, cubed
2 tbsp lime juice
2 tbsp coconut cream
400g/14oz tinned chopped tomatoes
125g/4oz mangetout
1 onion, chopped
2 red (bell) peppers sliced
1 tsp each cayenne pepper, tumeric & garlic salt
300g/11oz fine egg noodles
Low cal cooking oil spray
Salt & pepper to taste

Method:

• Preheat the oven to 200C/400F/Gas Mark 6
• Gently sauté the fish, peppers, mangetout, spices and onions in a frying pan with a little low cal spray for a few minutes.
• Add the chopped tomatoes & coconut cream and warm through.
• Meanwhile cook the noodles in salted boing water until tender. Drain and place in an ovenproof dish along with all the other ingredients, except the lime juice.
• Season, cover and cook for 30-40 minutes or until everything is piping hot.
• Stir through the lime juice and serve.

The coconut cream gives this dish a lovely creaminess but you could use low fat coconut milk if you wanted to cut down on the calories even more.

58

Haddock & Bamboo Shoot Fish Stew

Serves 4

Method:

• Preheat the oven to 200C/400F/Gas Mark 6
• Place the corn flour, five spice powder and haddock into a plastic bag and shake to give the fish a good flour covering.
• Sauté the floured fish, peppers, mangetout, garlic and onions in a frying pan with a little low cal spray for a few minutes.
• Meanwhile cook the noodles in salted boing water until tender. Drain and place in an ovenproof dish along with all the other ingredients.
• Season, cover and cook for 30-40 minutes or until everything is piping hot.
• Adjust the seasoning and serve.

Chinese five-spice is a classic spice combination. Try this with plenty of soy sauce to serve.

Ingredients:

500g/1lb 2oz skinless, boneless haddock fillets, cubed
1 tbsp corn flour
2 tsp Chinese five-spice powder
150g/5oz ready to eat bamboo shoots, drained
Bunch spring onions/ scallions, chopped
2 garlic cloves, crushed
1 tbsp lime juice
400g/14oz tinned chopped tomatoes
125g/4oz mangetout
1 onion, chopped
2 tbsp soy sauce
2 red (bell) peppers, sliced
300g/11oz fine egg noodles
Low cal cooking oil spray
Salt & pepper to taste

Lemon, Olive & Fish One Pot
Serves 4

350 CALORIES PER SERVING

Ingredients:

600g/1lb 5oz white meaty skinless, boneless fish fillets, cut into large cubes
250g/9oz tinned chickpeas, drained
250g/9oz vine ripened tomatoes, finely chopped
125g/4oz French beans, whole
2 tbsp plain/all purpose flour
1 tsp each ground cumin, turmeric and coriander/cilantro
2 garlic cloves, crushed
½ lemon, cut into thin slices
2 tbsp pine nuts
50g/2oz pitted black olives
3 tbsp freshly chopped coriander/cilantro
60ml/ ¼ cup fish stock/broth
Low cal cooking oil spray
Salt & pepper to taste

Method:

• Preheat the oven to 180C/350F/Gas Mark 5.
• Place the cubed fish in a plastic bag with the flour and shake well to cover the cubes.
• Quickly seal the fish in a frying pan with a little low cal spray for a minute or two on a high heat.
• Combine all the ingredients, except the chopped coriander in an ovenproof dish.
• Season, cover and cook in the oven for 30-40 minutes or until the fish is cooked through and piping hot.
• Sprinkle with chopped coriander and serve.

Any firm white fish fillets will work fine with this recipe. Season the fish well before coating in flour.

Italian Tuna Stew
Serves 4

Method:

• Preheat the oven to 180C/350F/Gas Mark 5.
• Season the tuna cubes and quickly seal in a frying pan with a little low cal spray for a minute or two on a high heat.
• Combine all the ingredients in an ovenproof dish. Cover and cook in the oven for 30-40 minutes or until the fish is cooked through and piping hot.
• Season and serve.

Ingredients:

700g/1lb 9oz fresh tuna steaks, cut into large cubes
600g/1lb 5oz vine ripened tomatoes, finely chopped
125g/4oz mangetout
2 garlic cloves, crushed
200g/7oz courgette/zuchinni, sliced
2 tbsp each freshly chopped oregano & basil
2 tbsp tomato puree/paste
60ml/¼ cup fish stock/broth
1 tsp brown sugar
Low cal cooking oil spray
Salt & pepper to taste

Fresh tuna steak is a beautiful fish to cook with. If you prefer your tuna a little rare in the centre do not add the fish to the oven until 6-8 minutes before the end of cooking time.

Moroccan Sea Bass & Greens
Serves 4

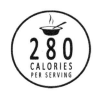

280 CALORIES PER SERVING

Ingredients:

600g/1lb 5oz skinless, boneless sea bass fillets
1 garlic clove, crushed
2 red peppers, sliced
400g/14oz tinned chopped tomatoes
1 tbsp each ground cumin & paprika
400g/14oz tinned chopped tomatoes
1 red chilli, deseeded and finely chopped
200g/7oz fresh spring greens, shredded
1 lemon, cut into wedges
60ml/¼ cup vegetable stock/broth
4 tbsp freshly chopped flat leaf parsley
Low cal cooking oil spray
Salt & pepper to taste

Method:

• Preheat the oven to 180C/350F/Gas Mark 5.
• Gently sauté the peppers, garlic and chillies in a frying pan with a little low cal spray for a few minutes.
• Carefully combine all the ingredients, except the chopped parsley and lemon wedges in an ovenproof dish. Season, cover and cook for 30-40 minutes or until the fish is cooked through and the vegetables are tender.
• Serve with chopped parsley sprinkled over the top and lemon wedges on the side.

Ready-to-cook shredded mixed spring greens are available almost everywhere. Chopped kale, cabbage or young spinach are all fine if that's what you have to hand.

320
CALORIES
PER SERVING

Cod Steaks, Asparagus & Split Lentils

Serves 4

Method:

- Preheat the oven to 180C/350F/Gas Mark 5.
- First simmer the lentils in boiling water for 15 minutes or until tender.
- Gently sauté the onions and garlic in a frying pan with a little low cal spray for a few minutes.
- First place the cod steaks into an ovenproof dish and cover with all the other ingredients, except the chopped coriander, lemons, asparagus and peas.
- Season, cover and cook in the oven for 20 minutes.
- Add the peas and asparagus tips to the dish, cover and cook for a further 20-30 minutes or until the cod is cooked through and the vegetables & lentils are tender.
- Add a little more stock or water during cooking if needed.
- Serve with chopped coriander sprinkled over the top and lemon wedges on the side.

Tenderstem broccoli spears rather than asparagus tips will work well in this recipe too.

Ingredients:

4 cod steaks, each weighing aprox 175g/6oz
175g/6oz red lentils
200g/7oz asparagus tips
2 garlic cloves, crushed
1 onion, chopped
1 tsp each ground ginger, turmeric and cumin
½ tsp cayenne pepper
2 limes, cut into wedges
3 tbsp freshly chopped coriander/cilantro
120ml/½ cup fish stock/ broth
125g/4oz peas
Low cal cooking oil spray
Salt & pepper to taste

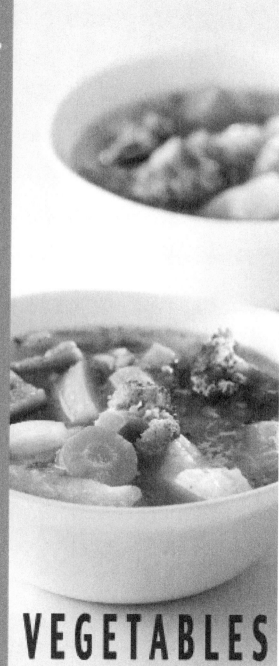

Skinny
WINTER

WARMERS

Soups, Stews
Casseroles &
One Pot Meals
Under 300, 400
& 500 calories

VEGETABLES

Greek Vegetable Moussaka
Serves 4

350 CALORIES PER SERVING

Ingredients:

2 aubergines/egg plant, sliced
1 tbsp crushed sea salt
75g/3oz red lentils, pre-soaked and ready to use
2 onions, chopped
380g/1½ cups vegetable stock/broth
2 garlic cloves, crushed
4 large portabella mushrooms, sliced
300g/11oz tinned chickpeas, drained
400g/14oz tinned chopped tomatoes
125g/4oz spinach leaves
2 tsp dried mixed herbs
3 tbsp freshly chopped basil
250ml/1 cup fat free Greek yoghurt
2 free range eggs
2 tsp grated parmesan cheese, or vegetarian alternative
Low cal cooking oil spray
Salt & pepper to taste

Method:

• Preheat the oven to 180C/350F/Gas Mark 5.
• Lay the aubergine slices out in a single layer and use the sea salt to sprinkle over them. Leave for 30-40 minutes whilst the salt works on tenderising the aubergine.
• Rinse the slices and sauté in a frying pan with a little low cal spray for a few minutes.
• Meanwhile beat together the eggs, grated parmesan and yoghurt. Set to one side will you combine all the other ingredients, except the chopped basil, into an ovenproof dish.
• Season, pour the yoghurt mix over the top and cook for 1hr – 1 ¼ hrs or until the vegetables are all tender and piping hot.
• Serve with the chopped basil sprinkled over the top.

Feel free to alter the balance of vegetables to use up whatever you have to hand.

420
CALORIES
PER SERVING

Spinach & Macaroni Double Cheese Bake
Serves 4

Method:

• Preheat the oven to 200C/400F/Gas Mark 6.
• Cook the pasta in salted boiling water until tender.
• Meanwhile gently warm through the mustard, crème fraiche, milk, nutmeg and cheeses in a saucepan.
• Combine all the ingredients in an ovenproof dish.
• Season well, cover and place in the oven for 25-30 minutes or until piping hot.

Ingredients:

400g/14oz macaroni pasta
2 tbsp dijon mustard
250ml/1 cup low fat crème fraiche
6 tbsp milk
½ tsp nutmeg
200g/7oz grated mature cheddar cheese
100g/7oz grated double gloucester cheese
125g/4oz spinach, chopped
Salt & pepper to taste

Use vegetarian alternative cheeses if you wish to make this extra cheesy macaroni bake.

Mixed Bean & Fresh Chive Chilli
Serves 4

Ingredients:

2 red onions, sliced
400g/14oz tinned chopped tomatoes
800g/1 ¾lb tinned mixed beans
4 tbsp tomato puree/paste
125g/4oz button mushrooms, sliced
3 carrots, finely chopped
1 tsp each ground chilli powder, cumin, paprika & coriander/cilantro
3 garlic cloves, crushed
2 tsp brown sugar
6 tbsp freshly chopped chives
4 tbsp sour cream
Low cal cooking oil spray
Salt & pepper to taste

Method:

• Preheat the oven to 200C/400F/Gas Mark 6.
• Gently sauté the onion, garlic and mushrooms in a little low cal oil until softened.
• Combine all the ingredients, except the chopped chives and sour cream, in an ovenproof dish.
• Season well, cover and cook for 30-35 minutes or until piping hot.
• Place in four bowls with a dollop of sour cream in the middle of each and the chopped chives sprinkled over the top.

Greek yoghurt will do just as well as sour cream in this recipe.

380 CALORIES PER SERVING

Spinach & Beans
Serves 4

Method:

• Preheat the oven to 180C/350F/Gas Mark 5.
• Gently sauté the onions, tomatoes, and garlic in a frying pan with a little low cal spray for a few minutes.
• Combine all the ingredients, except the pine nuts, in an ovenproof dish.
• Season, cover and cook for 30-40 minutes or until the vegetables are all tender and piping hot.
• Meanwhile toast the pine nuts in a dry pan for a few minutes.
• Season the vegetables and serve with the pine nuts sprinkled over the top.

Ingredients:

400g/14oz haricot beans, drained
400g/14oz spinach leaves
400g/14oz vine ripened tomatoes, cut into wedges
1 tsp each cumin and paprika
2 onions, chopped
2 tbsp raisins, chopped
60ml/ ¼ cup vegetable stock/broth
2 garlic cloves, crushed
2 tbsp pine nuts
Low cal cooking oil spray
Salt & pepper to taste

Be careful not to burn the pine nuts when you toast them. A medium heat under a dry pan will be enough to gently brown them.

Leek & Sundried Tomatoes
Serves 4

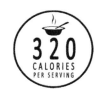

3 2 0
CALORIES
PER SERVING

Ingredients:

6 leeks, chopped
400g/14oz courgettes/
zuchinni, diced
60g/2oz sundried
tomatoes, chopped
60g/2oz pitted olives,
chopped
200g/7oz baby corn sliced
lengthways in half
1 garlic clove, crushed
1 tbsp soy sauce
75g/3oz puy lentils, pre-
soaked and ready to use
120ml/ ½ cup vegetable
stock/broth
4 tbsp freshly chopped flat
leaf parsley
Low cal cooking oil spray
Salt & pepper to taste

Method:

• Preheat the oven to 180C/350F/Gas Mark 5.
• Gently sauté the leeks, courgettes and garlic in a frying pan with a little low cal spray for a few minutes.
• Combine all the ingredients, except the chopped parsley in an ovenproof dish.
• Season, cover and cook for 30-40 minutes or until the vegetables are all tender and piping hot.
• Serve with the parsley sprinkled over the top.

This is a really simple light suppertime meal. Feel free to add a little more soy sauce to the dish when serving if you like.

Traditional Daal & Coconut Milk
Serves 4

Method:

- Preheat the oven to 180C/350F/Gas Mark 5.
- Combine all the ingredients, except the almonds, chopped coriander, limes and yoghurt in an ovenproof dish.
- Season, cover and cook for 50-60 minutes or until the lentils are tender.
- Add a little more stock during cooking if needed.
- Serve with the coriander and almonds sprinkled over the top and lime wedges and yoghurt on the side.

Ingredients:

300g/11oz red lentils
150g/5oz vine ripened tomatoes, chopped
2 carrots, finely chopped
3 garlic cloves, crushed
1 tsp each ground turmeric, coriander/cilantro, cumin, garam masala, ginger & chilli powder
½ tsp brown sugar
250ml/1 cup vegetable stock/broth
250ml/1 cup low fat coconut milk
2 limes, cut into wedges
4 tbsp freshly chopped coriander/cilantro
4 tbsp fat free Greek yoghurt
1 tbsp ground almonds
Salt & pepper to taste

Daal is one of the most important staples of Indian, Nepali, Pakistani and Bangladeshi cuisine.

Eastern Spiced Vegetables
Serves 4

240 CALORIES PER SERVING

Ingredients:

400g/14oz tinned chickpeas, drained
400g/14oz tinned chopped tomatoes
150g/5oz courgettes/ zuchinni, sliced
1 red onion, sliced
3 carrots, chopped
2 celery sticks, chopped
2 garlic cloves, crushed
1 tsp each ground coriander/cilantro, cumin & crushed chilli flakes
½ tsp ground cinnamon
60ml/¼ cup vegetable stock/broth
4 tbsp freshly chopped mint
Low cal cooking oil spray
Salt & pepper to taste

Method:

• Preheat the oven to 180C/350F/Gas Mark 5.
• Gently sauté the courgettes, onions, carrots, celery and garlic in a frying pan with a little low cal spray for a few minutes
• Combine all the ingredients, except the chopped mint in an ovenproof dish.
• Season, cover and cook for 30-40 minutes or until the vegetables are tender and piping hot.
• Serve with chopped mint sprinkled over the top.

Adjust the quantity of chilli flakes in this recipe to suit your own taste.

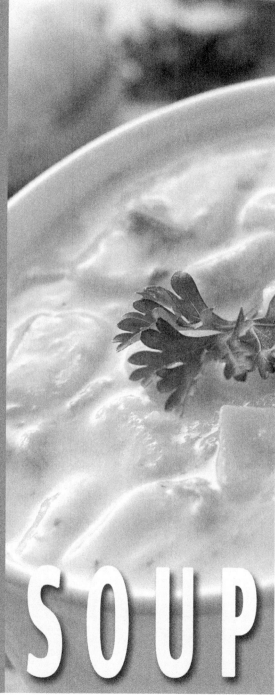

Skinny WINTER

WARMERS

Soups, Stews
Casseroles &
One Pot Meals
Under 300, 400
& 500 calories

SOUP

Mexican Black-Eyed Bean Soup

Serves 4

180 CALORIES PER SERVING

Ingredients:

1 tbsp olive oil
2 garlic cloves, crushed
1 red chilli, deseeded and chopped
1 red onion, chopped
250ml/1 cup vegetable stock/broth
250ml/1 cup tomato passata/sieved tomatoes
½ tsp each ground cumin, paprika & brown sugar
125g/4oz vine ripened tomatoes, chopped
200g/7oz tinned black eyed beans, rinsed
2 tbsp lime juice
3 tbsp freshly chopped coriander/cilantro
4 tbsp fat free Greek yoghurt
Salt & pepper to taste

Method:

• Gently sauté the onions, garlic and chilli in the olive oil for a few minutes until softened.
• Add all the ingredients, except the lime juice, chopped coriander and yoghurt, to a saucepan.
• Cover and leave to gently simmer for 20-30 minutes or until everything is tender and cooked through. Use a food processor or blender to blend to your preferred consistency.
• Stir through the lime juice, adjust the seasoning, sprinkle with chopped coriander and serve with a dollop of yoghurt.

This soup is best served as chunky as possible to keep the majority of the beans intact.

131
CALORIES
PER SERVING

Pea & Mint Soup
Serves 4

Method:

• Gently sauté the onions in the olive oil for a few minutes until softened.
• Add all the ingredients, except the fresh chopped herbs, to a saucepan.
• Cover and leave to gently simmer for 20-30 minutes or until everything is tender and cooked through.
• Use a food processor or blender to blend to your preferred consistency.
• Adjust the seasoning, sprinkle with chopped herbs and serve with a dollop of yoghurt.

Ingredients:

1 tbsp olive oil
1 onion, chopped
1 tsp dried thyme
750ml/3 cups vegetable stock/broth
400g/14oz peas
2 tbsp each freshly chopped flat leaf parsley & mint
Salt & pepper to taste

Fresh or frozen peas will work just as well in this recipe.

Creamy Mushroom Soup
Serves 4

170 CALORIES PER SERVING

Ingredients:

1 tbsp olive oil
1 leek, chopped
750ml/3 cups vegetable stock/broth
450g/1lb chestnut mushrooms, chopped
1 garlic clove, crushed
1 tbsp porcini mushrooms, rehydrated and chopped
120ml/½ cup single cream
½ tsp dried thyme
¼ tsp ground nutmeg
2 tbsp finely chopped chives, to serve

Method:

• First place the dried porcini mushrooms in a little warm water for 10 minutes. Chop and gently sauté with the leeks and chestnut mushrooms in the olive oil for a few minutes until softened.
• Add all the ingredients, except the cream and chives, to a saucepan. Cover and leave to gently simmer for 20-30 minutes or until everything is tender and cooked through.
• Use a food processor or blender to blend to your preferred consistency.
• Adjust the seasoning, add a swirl of cream to each bowl, sprinkle with chives and serve.

Experiment with whichever type of mushrooms you prefer or have to hand.

Ginger & Parsnip Soup
Serves 4

Method:

• Gently sauté the onions in the olive oil for a few minutes until softened.
• Add all the ingredients to a saucepan. Cover and leave to gently simmer for 20-30 minutes or until everything is tender and cooked through.
• Use a food processor or blender to blend to your preferred consistency.
• Adjust the seasoning and serve.

Ingredients:

1 tbsp olive oil
1 onion, chopped
4 garlic cloves, crushed
1 tbsp freshly grated ginger
½ tsp each ground cumin & paprika
500g/1lb 2oz parsnips, peeled & chopped
500ml/2 cups vegetable stock/broth
250ml/1 cup semi skimmed milk
Salt & pepper to taste

You could add more milk and less stock if you wanted a creamier consistency.

Chickpea & Coriander Soup

Serves 4

144 CALORIES PER SERVING

Ingredients:

1 tbsp olive oil
300g/11oz tinned chickpeas, drained
1 red chilli, deseeded and chopped
2 tsp cumin seeds, crushed with a pestle & mortar
4 tsp freshly chopped coriander/cilantro
4 cloves garlic, crushed
1 tsp ground turmeric
750ml/3 cups vegetable stock/broth
Zest of 1 lemon
2 tbsp lemon juice
Salt & pepper to taste

Method:

• Add all the ingredients to a saucepan, except the lemon juice and chopped coriander/cilantro.
• Cover and leave to gently simmer for 20-30 minutes or until everything is tender and cooked through.
• Use a food processor or blender to blend to your preferred consistency.
• Add the lemon juice, adjust the seasoning, sprinkle with coriander and serve.

Stirring through the lemon juice just before serving really 'lifts' this earthy soup.

170 CALORIES PER SERVING

Warming Celery & Potato Soup
Serves 4

Method:

• Gently sauté the chopped leeks in the olive oil for a few minutes until softened.
• Add all the ingredients, except the cream, to a saucepan. Cover and leave to gently simmer for 20-30 minutes or until everything is tender and cooked through.
• Use a food processor or blender to blend to your preferred consistency.
• Stir through the cream and leave to warm for minute or two.
• Adjust the seasoning and serve.

Ingredients:

1 tbsp olive oil
350g/12oz celery stalks, chopped
125g/4oz potatoes, peeled and cubed
1 leek, chopped
250ml/1 cup vegetable stock/broth
1 tsp ground cumin
½ tsp celery seeds
250ml/1 cup whole milk
250ml/1 cup single cream
Salt & pepper to taste

This is a really fresh, creamy soup which is fantastic on a cold day.

Classic Cauliflower & Stilton Soup

Serves 4

220
CALORIES
PER SERVING

Ingredients:

1 tbsp olive oil
1 onion, chopped
750ml/3 cups vegetable
stock/broth
1 stick celery, chopped
1 leek, chopped
125g/4oz potatoes, peeled
& cubed
1 bay leaf (remove before
blending)
450g/1lb cauliflower
florets
120ml/½ cup single cream
50g/2oz stilton cheese
2 tbsp freshly chopped
chives
Salt & pepper to taste

Method:

• Gently sauté the chopped leeks and onions in the olive oil for a few minutes until softened.
• Add all the ingredients, except the cream and chives, to a saucepan. Cover and leave to gently simmer for 20-30 minutes or until everything is tender and cooked through.
• Use a food processor or blender to blend to your preferred consistency.
• Stir through the cream and leave to warm for minute or two.
• Adjust the seasoning and serve with the chopped chives sprinkled on top.

The stilton cheese in this recipe can be substituted for extra mature cheddar if you prefer.

Italian Pasta Soup
Serves 4

Method:

• Gently sauté the chopped onions in the olive oil for a few minutes until softened.
• Add all the ingredients to a saucepan, except the grated parmesan cheese. Cover and leave to gently simmer for 20-30 minutes or until everything is tender and cooked through. \
• Use a food processor or blender to blend to your preferred consistency.
• Adjust the seasoning, sprinkle with parmesan and serve.

Ingredients:

1 tbsp olive oil
225g/8oz tinned Italian beans eg. borlotti or cannellini
125g/4oz soup pasta
1 tsp dried rosemary
3 garlic cloves, crushed
2 tbsp tomato puree/paste
1 onion, chopped
1 tbsp freshly grated parmesan cheese
750ml/3 cups vegetable stock/broth
Salt & pepper to taste

Use any type of really small pasta shape you like for this recipe. It's best served as chunky as possible to keep the pasta shapes intact.

Spicy Carrot & Honey Soup

Serves 4

Ingredients:

1 tbsp olive oil
2 leeks, sliced
650g/1lb 7oz carrots, chopped
2 tsp clear runny honey
1 bay leaf (remove before blending)
1 tsp crushed chilli flakes
750ml/3 cups vegetable stock/broth
Salt & pepper to taste

Method:

• Gently sauté the chopped leeks in the olive oil for a few minutes until softened.
• Add all the ingredients to a saucepan. Cover and leave to gently simmer for 20-30 minutes or until everything is tender and cooked through.
• Remove the bay leaf and use a food processor or blender to blend to your preferred consistency.
• Adjust the seasoning and serve.

Adjust the crushed chilli flake quantities to suit your own taste.

Pumpkin Soup

Serves 4

Method:

• Add all the ingredients to a saucepan, except the pumpkin seeds and cream.

• Cover and leave to gently simmer for 20-30 minutes or until everything is tender and cooked through. Use a food processor or blender to blend to your preferred consistency.

• Stir through the cream and leave to warm for a minute or two.

• Adjust the seasoning and serve with the pumpkin seeds sprinkled on top.

Ingredients:

1 tbsp olive oil
1 tbsp dried pumpkin seeds, chopped
450g/1lb pumpkin flesh, peeled and cubed
200g/7oz potatoes, peeled and cubed
750ml/3 cups vegetable stock/broth
60ml/ ½ cup single cream
Salt & pepper to taste

You could substitute any kind of edible chopped seeds or nuts to sprinkle on top of the soup.

Chicken & Broccoli Noodle Soup

Serves 4

230 CALORIES PER SERVING

Ingredients:

1 tbsp olive oil

125g/4oz fresh tenderstem broccoli spears, roughly chopped

500ml/2 cups chicken stock/broth

250ml/1 cup dry white wine

2 garlic cloves, crushed

1 tsp each freshly chopped flat leaf parsley & dill

350g/12oz skinless chicken breast, chopped

50g/2oz rice noodles

1 leek, chopped

1 onion, chopped

Salt & pepper to taste

Method:

• Gently sauté the chicken, onions and leeks in the olive oil for a few minutes.

• Add all the ingredients to a saucepan. Cover and leave to gently simmer for 20-30 minutes or until everything is tender and cooked through.

• Use a food processor or blender to blend to your preferred consistency.

• Adjust the seasoning and serve.

Use ordinary broccoli if you can't get tenderstem or purple sprouting broccoli spears.

185
CALORIES
PER SERVING

Spelt Barley & Sirloin Soup
Serves 4

Method:

• Gently sauté the steak, onions and leeks in the olive oil for a few minutes.
• Add all the ingredients to a saucepan. Cover and leave to gently simmer for 20-30 minutes or until everything is tender and cooked through.
• Use a food processor or blender to blend to your preferred consistency.
• Adjust the seasoning and serve.

Ingredients:

1 tbsp olive oil
225g/8oz lean sirloin steak, chopped
2 tsp dried mixed herbs
50g/2oz pre-soaked spelt barley
1 carrot, chopped
1 onion, chopped
1 leek, chopped
2 celery stalks, chopped
750ml/3 cups beef stock/broth
Salt & pepper to taste

Feel free to use a less expensive cut of beef for the soup if you like, it will still taste good!

Thai Chicken Soup
Serves 4

290 CALORIES PER SERVING

Ingredients:

1 tsp olive oil
200g/7oz skinless chicken breast
250ml/1 cup reduced fat coconut milk
500ml/2 cups chicken stock/broth
2 stalks fresh lemon grass, peeled & finely chopped
1 bunch spring onion/ scallions, chopped
2 tbsp lime juice
1 tsp freshly grated ginger
1 tbsp soy sauce
1 tsp ground ginger
1 red chilli, deseeded and finely chopped
1 tbsp corn flour dissolved into a little warm water to form a paste
Salt & pepper to taste

Method:

• Gently sauté the chicken in the olive oil for a few minutes.
• Add all the ingredients, except the coconut milk and lime juice, to a saucepan. Cover and leave to gently simmer for 20-30 minutes or until everything is tender and cooked through.
• Use a food processor or blender to blend to your preferred consistency.
• Add the coconut milk, stir and leave to warm through for 2-3 minutes.
• Adjust the seasoning, add the lime juice and serve.

This Thai soup is a great combination of citrus flavours and robust spices.

290
CALORIES
PER SERVING

Chicken & Split Pea Broth
Serves 4

Method:

• Gently sauté the chicken, leeks and chopped onions in the olive oil for a few minutes.
• Add all the ingredients to a saucepan. Cover and leave to gently simmer for 20-30 minutes or until everything is tender and cooked through.
• Use a food processor or blender to blend to your preferred consistency.
• Adjust the seasoning and serve.

Ingredients:

1 tbsp olive oil
225g/8oz skinless chicken breast
50g/2oz pre-soaked yellow split peas
750ml/3 cups chicken stock/broth
1 carrot, chopped
1 onion, chopped
1 leek, chopped
50g/2oz pearl barley
1 tsp freshly chopped thyme
2 stalks celery, chopped
Salt & pepper to taste

Avoid blending this soup too much. It's best served chunky.

Pancetta & Lentil Soup
Serves 4

230
CALORIES
PER SERVING

Ingredients:

1 tbsp olive oil
1 onion, chopped
2 garlic cloves, crushed
150g/5oz pancetta cubes
200g/7oz red lentils
750ml/3 cups chicken
stock/broth
3 fresh tomatoes, chopped
2 bay leaves (remove
before blending)
¼ tsp ground all spice
125g/4oz potatoes, peeled
& cubed
Bunch spring onions/
scallions, chopped
4 tbsp freshly chopped flat
leaf parsley
Salt & pepper to taste

Method:

• Gently sauté the pancetta and chopped onions in the olive oil for a few minutes.
• Add all the ingredients, except the chopped parsley, to a saucepan. Cover and leave to gently simmer for 20-30 minutes or until everything is tender and cooked through.
• Remove the bay leaves. Use a food processor or blender to blend to your preferred consistency.
• Adjust the seasoning, sprinkle with parsley and serve.

Serve with a swirl of single cream if you want a more luxurious texture.

Kale & Chorizo Soup
Serves 4

Method:

- Gently sauté the onions, chorizo and garlic in the olive oil for a few minutes.
- Add all the ingredients to a saucepan. Cover and leave to gently simmer for 20-30 minutes or until everything is tender and cooked through.
- Use a food processor or blender to blend to your preferred consistency.
- Adjust the seasoning and serve.

Ingredients:

1 tbsp olive oil
175g/6oz kale, shredded
2 onions, chopped
4 garlic cloves, crushed
125g/4oz cooking chorizo sausages, sliced
150g/5oz potatoes, peeled & cubed
750ml/3 cups chicken stock/broth
Salt & pepper to taste

Use raw chorizo sausages rather than the more widely available cured chorizo sausage.

Pork & Ginger Soup
Serves 4

215 CALORIES PER SERVING

Ingredients:

1 tbsp olive oil
1 onion, chopped
3 garlic cloves, crushed
1 tsp fish sauce
1 red chilli, deseeded and finely chopped
250g/9oz pork tenderloin, thinly sliced
100g/3½oz long grain rice
750ml/3 cups chicken stock/broth
2 tsp freshly grated ginger
Small bunch spring onions/scallions, sliced lengthways
Salt & pepper to taste

Method:

• Gently sauté the onions and pork in the olive oil for a few minutes.
• Add all the ingredients, except the chopped spring onions, to a saucepan.
• Cover and leave to gently simmer for 20-30 minutes or until everything is tender and cooked through.
• Use a food processor or blender to blend to your preferred consistency.
• Adjust the seasoning, sprinkle with springs onions and serve.

Soft noodles are a great alternative to this recipe instead of rice.

Ham & Kidney Bean Soup
Serves 4

Method:

- Add all the ingredients to a saucepan.
- Cover and leave to gently simmer for 20-30 minutes or until everything is tender and cooked through.
- Use a food processor or blender to blend to your preferred consistency.
- Adjust the seasoning and serve.

Ingredients:

200g/7oz tinned red kidney beans
150g/5oz smoked ham, chopped
125g/4oz potatoes, peeled & cubed
1 parsnip, peeled & chopped
750ml/3 cups chicken stock/broth
2 garlic cloves, crushed
125g/4oz tenderstem broccoli, roughly chopped
Salt & pepper to taste

Any kind of cured pork meat will work well in this recipe, try cooked bacon or gammon but be careful with the seasoning as you don't want the soup to be too salty.

Saffron & Fennel Seafood Soup

Serves 4

Ingredients:

1 tbsp olive oil
3 garlic cloves, crushed
1 onion, chopped
Half a fennel bulb, chopped
250g/9oz skinless, boneless white fish fillet, chopped
125g/4oz shelled cooked prawns
Large pinch saffron threads
½ tsp crushed chilli flakes
750ml/3 cups chicken stock/broth
1 fresh tomato, chopped
3 tbsp each tomato puree/paste & freshly chopped flat leaf parsley
Zest of 1 orange
Salt & pepper to taste

Method:

• Gently sauté the onions in the olive oil for a few minutes.
• Add all the ingredients, except the chopped parsley, to a saucepan.
• Cover and leave to gently simmer for 20-30 minutes or until everything is tender and cooked through.
• Use a food processor or blender to blend to your preferred consistency.
• Adjust the seasoning, sprinkle with parsley and serve.

Don't chop the fish too small, instead leave it in reasonably large chunks and barely blend.

290
CALORIES
PER SERVING

Spiced Prawn & Rice Soup
Serves 4

Method:

• Gently sauté the onions in the olive oil for a few minutes.
• Add all the ingredients to a saucepan. Cover and leave to gently simmer for 20-30 minutes or until everything is tender and cooked through.
• Use a food processor or blender to blend to your preferred consistency.
• Adjust the seasoning and serve.

Ingredients:

1 tbsp olive oil
2 garlic cloves, crushed
200g/7oz peeled cooked prawns
1 onion, chopped
75g/3oz basmati rice
2 fresh tomatoes, chopped
750ml/3 cups fish stock/broth
1 tsp each ground turmeric, cumin, chilli powder & coriander/cilantro
2 tbsp coconut cream
Salt & pepper to taste

This soup can be served as a main course when paired with chapatti or roti flat bread.

CONVERSION CHART: DRY INGREDIENTS

Metric	Imperial
7g	¼ oz
15g	½ oz
20g	¾ oz
25g	1 oz
40g	1½oz
50g	2oz
60g	2½oz
75g	3oz
100g	3½oz
125g	4oz
140g	4½oz
150g	5oz
165g	5½oz
175g	6oz
200g	7oz
225g	8oz
250g	9oz
275g	10oz
300g	11oz
350g	12oz
375g	13oz
400g	14oz

Metric	Imperial
425g	15oz
450g	1lb
500g	1lb 2oz
550g	1¼lb
600g	1lb 5oz
650g	1lb 7oz
675g	1½lb
700g	1lb 9oz
750g	1lb 11oz
800g	1¾lb
900g	2lb
1kg	2¼lb
1.1kg	2½lb
1.25kg	2¾lb
1.35kg	3lb
1.5kg	3lb 6oz
1.8kg	4lb
2kg	4½lb
2.25kg	5lb
2.5kg	5½lb
2.75kg	6lb

CONVERSION CHART: LIQUID MEASURES

Metric	Imperial	US
25ml	1fl oz	
60ml	2fl oz	¼ cup
75ml	2½ fl oz	
100ml	3½fl oz	
120ml	4fl oz	½ cup
150ml	5fl oz	
175ml	6fl oz	
200ml	7fl oz	
250ml	8½ fl oz	1 cup
300ml	10½ fl oz	
360ml	12½ fl oz	
400ml	14fl oz	
450ml	15½ fl oz	
600ml	1 pint	
750ml	1¼ pint	3 cups
1 litre	1½ pints	4 cups

Other
COOKNATION
TITLES

If you enjoyed 'Skinny Winter Warmers' we'd really appreciate your feedback. Reviews help others decide if this is the right book for them so a moment of your time would be appreciated.

Thank you.

You may also be interested in other '**Skinny**' titles in the CookNation series. You can find all the following great titles by searching under '**CookNation**'.

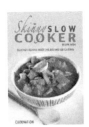

The Skinny Slow Cooker Recipe Book

Delicious Recipes Under 300, 400 And 500 Calories.

Paperback / eBook

More Skinny Slow Cooker Recipes

75 More Delicious Recipes Under 300, 400 & 500 Calories.

Paperback / eBook

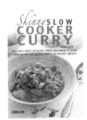

The Skinny Slow Cooker Curry Recipe Book

Low Calorie Curries From Around The World

Paperback / eBook

The Skinny Slow Cooker Soup Recipe Book

Simple, Healthy & Delicious Low Calorie Soup Recipes For Your Slow Cooker. All Under 100, 200 & 300 Calories.

Paperback / eBook

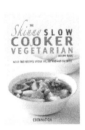

The Skinny Slow Cooker Vegetarian Recipe Book

40 Delicious Recipes Under 200, 300 And 400 Calories.

Paperback / eBook

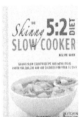

The Skinny 5:2 Slow Cooker Recipe Book

Skinny Slow Cooker Recipe And Menu Ideas Under 100, 200, 300 & 400 Calories For Your 5:2 Diet.

Paperback / eBook

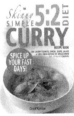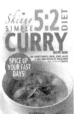

The Skinny 5:2 Curry Recipe Book

Spice Up Your Fast Days With Simple Low Calorie Curries, Snacks, Soups, Salads & Sides Under 200, 300 & 400 Calories

Paperback / eBook

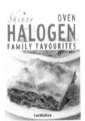

The Skinny Halogen Oven Family Favourites Recipe Book

Healthy, Low Calorie Family Meal-Time Halogen Oven Recipes Under 300, 400 and 500 Calories

Paperback / eBook

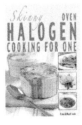

Skinny Halogen Oven Cooking For One

Single Serving, Healthy, Low Calorie Halogen Oven Recipes Under 200, 300 and 400 Calories

Paperback / eBook

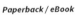

Skinny Winter Warmers Recipe Book

Soups, Stews, Casseroles & One Pot Meals Under 300, 400 & 500 Calories.

Paperback / eBook

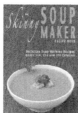

The Skinny Soup Maker Recipe Book

Delicious Low Calorie, Healthy and Simple Soup Recipes Under 100, 200 and 300 Calories. Perfect For Any Diet and Weight Loss Plan.

Paperback / eBook

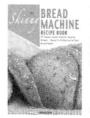

The Skinny Bread Machine Recipe Book

70 Simple, Lower Calorie, Healthy Breads...Baked To Perfection In Your Bread Maker.

Paperback / eBook

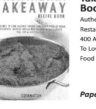

The Skinny Indian Takeaway Recipe Book

Authentic British Indian Restaurant Dishes Under 300, 400 And 500 Calories. The Secret To Low Calorie Indian Takeaway Food At Home

Paperback / eBook

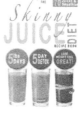

The Skinny Juice Diet Recipe Book

5lbs, 5 Days. The Ultimate Kick-Start Diet and Detox Plan to Lose Weight & Feel Great!

Paperback / eBook

The Skinny 5:2 Diet Recipe Book Collection

All The 5:2 Fast Diet Recipes You'll Ever Need. All Under 100, 200, 300, 400 And 500 Calories

Available only on eBook

eBook

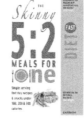

The Skinny 5:2 Fast Diet Meals For One

Single Serving Fast Day Recipes & Snacks Under 100, 200 & 300 Calories

Paperback / eBook

The Skinny 5:2 Fast Diet Vegetarian Meals For One

Single Serving Fast Day Recipes & Snacks Under 100, 200 & 300 Calories

Paperback / eBook

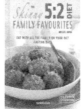

The Skinny 5:2 Fast Diet Family Favourites Recipe Book

Eat With All The Family On Your Diet Fasting Days

Paperback / eBook

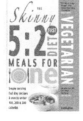

The Skinny 5:2 Fast Diet Family Favorites Recipe Book *U.S.A. EDITION*

Dine With All The Family On Your Diet Fasting Days

Available only on eBook

Paperback / eBook

The Skinny 5:2 Diet Chicken Dishes Recipe Book

Delicious Low Calorie Chicken Dishes Under 300, 400 & 500 Calories

Paperback / eBook

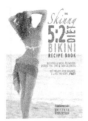

The Skinny 5:2 Bikini Diet Recipe Book

Recipes & Meal Planners Under 100, 200 & 300 Calories. Get Ready For Summer & Lose Weight...FAST!

Paperback / eBook

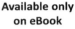

Available only on eBook

The Paleo Diet For Beginners Slow Cooker Recipe Book

Gluten Free, Everyday Essential Slow Cooker Paleo Recipes For Beginners

eBook

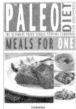

The Paleo Diet For Beginners Meals For One

The Ultimate Paleo Single Serving Cookbook

Paperback / eBook

Available only on eBook

The Paleo Diet For Beginners Holidays

Thanksgiving, Christmas & New Year Paleo Friendly Recipes

eBook

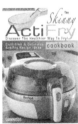

Available only on eBook

The Healthy Kids Smoothie Book

40 Delicious Goodness In A Glass Recipes for Happy Kids.

eBook

The Skinny Slow Cooker Summer Recipe Book

Fresh & Seasonal Summer Recipes For Your Slow Cooker. All Under 300, 400 And 500 Calories.

Paperback / eBook

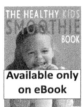

The Skinny ActiFry Cookbook

Guilt-free and Delicious ActiFry Recipe Ideas: Discover The Healthier Way to Fry!

Paperback / eBook

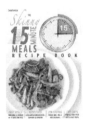

The Skinny 15 Minute Meals Recipe Book

Delicious, Nutritious & Super-Fast Meals in 15 Minutes Or Less. All Under 300, 400 & 500 Calories.

Paperback / eBook

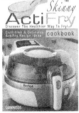

The Skinny Mediterranean Recipe Book

Simple, Healthy & Delicious Low Calorie Mediterranean Diet Dishes. All Under 200, 300 & 400 Calories.

Paperback / eBook

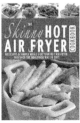

The Skinny Hot Air Fryer Cookbook

Delicious & Simple Meals For Your Hot Air Fryer: Discover The Healthier Way To Fry.

Paperback / eBook

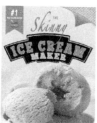

The Skinny Ice Cream Maker

Delicious Lower Fat, Lower Calorie Ice Cream, Frozen Yogurt & Sorbet Recipes For Your Ice Cream Maker

Paperback / eBook

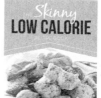

The Skinny Low Calorie Recipe Book

Great Tasting, Simple & Healthy Meals Under 300, 400 & 500 Calories. Perfect For Any Calorie Controlled Diet.

Paperback / eBook

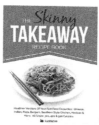

The Skinny Takeaway Recipe Book

Healthier Versions Of Your Fast Food Favourites: Chinese, Indian, Pizza, Burgers, Southern Style Chicken, Mexican & More. All Under 300, 400 & 500 Calories

Paperback / eBook

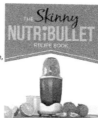

The Skinny Nutribullet Recipe Book

80+ Delicious & Nutritious Healthy Smoothie Recipes. Burn Fat, Lose Weight and Feel Great!

Paperback / eBook

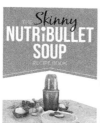

The Skinny Nutribullet Soup Recipe Book

Delicious, Quick & Easy, Single Serving Soups & Pasta Sauces For Your Nutribullet. All Under 100, 200, 300 & 400 Calories.

Paperback / eBook

Printed in Great Britain
by Amazon